DAVIS'S Compreh...

Laboratory & Diagnostic Tests with Nursing Implications

Activate your FREE subscription today!

You're two steps away from your **FREE**, 1-year subscription to **www.LabDxTest.com**, powered by Unbound Medicine.

powered by
unbound®
MEDICINE

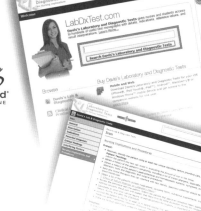

1. Simply type the following address into your web browser:

www.LabDxTest.com

2. Enter your unique, personal code printed on this page.

www.LabDxTest.com features all of the monographs from the **Davis's Comprehensive Handbook of Laboratory & Diagnostic Tests with Nursing Implications** database! It's accessible from your desktop, laptop, or any mobile device with a web browser.

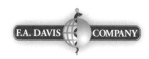

F.A. DAVIS COMPANY

5TH EDITION

Davis's

Comprehensive Handbook of
Laboratory
Diagnostic Tests with
Nursing Implications

Anne M. Van Leeuwen
Debra J. Poelhuis-Leth
Mickey Lynn Bladh

F. A. DAVIS COMPANY • Philadelphia

F.A. Davis Company
1915 Arch Street
Philadelphia, PA 19103

www.fadavis.com

Printed in the United States of America

Last digit indicates print number: 10 9 8 7 6 5 4 3

Publisher: Lisa B. Houck
Art and Design Manager: Carolyn O'Brien
Managing Editor: David Orzechowski
Project Editor: Victoria White
Digital Publishing Project Manager: Tyler Baber

As new scientific information becomes available through basic and clinical research, recommended treatments and drug therapies undergo changes. The authors and publisher have done everything possible to make this book accurate, up to date, and in accord with accepted standards at the time of publication. The authors, editors, and publisher are not responsible for errors or omissions or for consequences from application of the book, and make no warranty, expressed or implied, in regard to the contents of the book. Any practice described in this book should be applied by the reader in accordance with professional standards of care used in regard to the unique circumstances that may apply in each situation. The reader is advised always to check product information (package inserts) for changes and new information regarding dose and contraindications before administering any drug. Caution is especially urged when using new or infrequently ordered drugs.

Library of Congress Cataloging-in-Publication Data

Van Leeuwen, Anne M.
   Davis's comprehensive handbook of laboratory and diagnostic tests with nursing implications/Anne M. Van Leeuwen, Debra Poelhuis-Leth, Mickey Lynn Bladh.—5th ed.
       p. ; cm.
   Comprehensive handbook of laboratory & diagnostic tests with nursing implications
   Laboratory & diagnostic tests with nursing implications
   Rev. ed. of: Davis's comprehensive handbook of laboratory & diagnostic tests with nursing implications/Anne M. Van Leeuwen, Debra Poelhuis-Leth Mickey Lynn Bladh.
   Includes bibliographical references and index.
   ISBN 978-0-8036-3664-4
   I. Poelhuis-Leth, Debra J. II. Bladh, Mickey Lynn. III. Van Leeuwen, Anne M. Davis's comprehensive handbook of laboratory & diagnostic tests with nursing implications. IV. Title. V. Title: Comprehensive handbook of laboratory & diagnostic tests with nursing implications. VI. Title: Laboratory & diagnostic tests with nursing implications.
   [DNLM: 1. Clinical Laboratory Techniques—Handbooks. 2. Clinical Laboratory Techniques—Nurses' Instruction. 3. Nursing Diagnosis—methods. 4. Diagnostic Techniques and Procedures—Handbooks. 5. Diagnostic Techniques and Procedures—Nurses' Instruction. QY 39]

   616.07'5—dc23
                                          2012037821

Dedication

Inspiration springs from Passion. ... Passion is born from unconstrained love, commitment, and a vision no one else can own.

Lynda, thank you—I could not have done this without your love, strong support, and belief in me. My gratitude to Mom, Dad, Adele, Gram ... all my family and friends, for I am truly blessed by your humor and faith. A huge hug for my daughters, Sarah and Margaret—I love you very much. To my puppies, Maggie, Taylor, and Emma, for their endless and unconditional love. Many thanks to my friends and wonderful coauthors Debbie and Mickey; to all the folks at F.A. Davis, especially Rob, Victoria, and Cynthia for their guidance, support, and great ideas. And, very special thanks to Lisa Houck, publisher, for her friendship, excellent direction, and unwavering encouragement.

Anne M. Van Leeuwen, MA, BS, MT (ASCP)
Medical Laboratory Scientist
Sonora Quest Laboratories
Sun City West, Arizona

To Bill, my husband, who always shows his support for my professional endeavors. To my beautiful children, Abbie and Andy, I love you both; please remember to always push yourselves to excel. And to my parents for always showing pride in what I accomplished. Dad, I know you are still watching me from heaven and smiling. Lisa and Rob, your confidence, continued support, guidance, and assistance is always appreciated. Anne and Mickey, we are an awesome team, and I look forward to our continued friendship.

Debra J. Poelhuis-Leth, MS, RT, (R)(M)
Director, Radiology Program
Montgomery County Community College
Pottstown, Pennsylvania

An eternity of searching would never have provided me with a man more loving and supportive than my husband, Eric. He is the sunshine in my soul, and I will be forever grateful for the blessing of his presence in my life. I am grateful to my five children, Eric, Anni, Phillip, Mari, and Melissa, for the privilege of being their mom; always remember that you are limited only by your imagination and willingness to try. To Anne and Deb, thanks so much for the opportunity to spread my wings, for your patience and guidance, and thanks to Lynda for the miracle of finding me. To all of those at F.A. Davis—Rob, Victoria, and Lisa—you are the best. Lastly, to my beloved parents, thanks with hugs and kisses.

Mickey Lynn Bladh, RN, MSN
Coordinator, Nursing Education
Presbyterian Intercommunity Hospital
Whittier, California

About This Book

The authors would like to thank all the users of the previous editions for helping us identify what they like about this book as well as what might improve its value. We want to continue this dialogue. As writers, it is our desire to capture the interest of our readers, to provide essential information, and to continue to improve the presentation of the material in the book and ancillary products. We encourage our readers to provide feedback to the Web site and to the publisher's sales professionals. Your feedback helps us modify the material—to change with your changing needs. Several new monographs have been added: hepatitis E antibody, MRI venography, neonatal screening, procalcitonin, and US abdomen. Monographs have been expanded to include additional information; for example, we added new or updated information for more than 20 different tests related to topics in the main monographs including:

- Expanded material regarding genetic markers for Alzheimer's disease; tests used to diagnose gluten-sensitive enteropathies; immunosuppressant therapies used for organ transplant patients; genetic testing for drug resistance; description of the arterial brachial index; tests used to evaluate intermediate glycemic control; the use of pharmacogenetics to help explain why some patients don't respond as expected to their medications; and the use of home test kits
- Suggestions for patient teaching that reflect changes in standards of care, particularly with respect to cancer screening
- The most current Centers for Disease Control and Prevention (CDC) guidelines for communicable diseases such as syphilis, tuberculosis, and HIV
- The Institute of Medicine's most current national nutritional guidelines for all age groups
- The Critical Findings sections for lab and diagnostic studies include a sample statement that walks the nurse through the process for timely notification and documentation of critical values
- The Critical Findings sections are updated and enhanced to include conventional and SI units in the monographs as well as in the appendices that contain printable tables listing critical findings for diagnostic and laboratory studies
- The Critical Findings sections are updated and enhanced to include commonly reported pediatric and neonatal values for diagnostic and laboratory studies

Some monographs have been combined to consolidate similar tests, and a few less frequently used tests have been condensed into a mini-monograph format that highlights abbreviated test-specific facts, with the full monographs for those tests now resident on the DavisPlus Web site (http://davisplus.fadavis.com). The Reference Value heading in the laboratory monographs has been replaced with Normal Findings to (a) use terminology that is easier to recognize and interpret and (b) use consistent terminology in laboratory and diagnostic monographs. All of these changes have been made in response to feedback from our readers.

The authors have continued to enhance four areas in this new edition: pathophysiology that affects test results, patient safety, patient education, and integration of related laboratory and diagnostic testing. First, the Potential Diagnosis section includes an explanation of increased or decreased values, as many of you requested. We have added age-specific reference values for the neonatal, pediatric, and geriatric populations at the request of some of our readers. It should be mentioned that standardized information for the complexity of a geriatric population is difficult to document. Values may be increased or decreased in older adults due to the sole or combined effects of malnutrition, alcohol use, medications, and the presence of multiple chronic or acute diseases with or without muted symptoms. Second, the authors appreciate that nurses are the strongest patient advocates with a huge responsibility to protect the safety of their patients, and we have observed student nurses in clinical settings being interviewed by facility accreditation inspectors, so we have updated safety reminders, particularly with respect to positive patient identification, communication of critical information, proper timing of diagnostic procedures, rescheduling of specimen collection for therapeutic drug monitoring, use of evidence-based practices for prevention of surgical site infections, information regarding the move to track or limit exposure to radiation from CT studies for adults, and Image Gently guidelines for pediatric patients undergoing CT studies. The Pretest section reminds the nurse to positively identify the patient before providing care, treatment, or services. The Pretest section also addresses hand-off communication of critical information. The third area of emphasis coaches the student to focus on patient education and prepares the nurse to anticipate and respond to a patient's questions or concerns: describing the purpose of the procedure, addressing concerns about pain, understanding the implications of the test results, and describing post-procedural care. Various related Web sites for patient education are included throughout the book. And fourth, laboratory and diagnostic tests do not stand on their own—all the pieces fit together to form a picture. The section at the end of each monograph integrates both laboratory and diagnostic tests, providing a more complete picture of the studies that may be encountered in a patient's health-care experience. The authors thought it useful for a nurse to know what other tests might be ordered together—and all the related tests are listed alphabetically for ease of use.

Laboratory and diagnostic studies are essential components of a complete patient assessment. Examined in conjunction with an individual's history and physical examination, laboratory studies and diagnostic data provide clues about health status. Nurses are increasingly expected to integrate an understanding of laboratory and diagnostic procedures and expected outcomes in assessment, planning, implementation, and evaluation of nursing care. The data help develop and support nursing diagnoses, interventions, and outcomes.

Nurses may interface with laboratory and diagnostic testing on several levels, including:

- Interacting with patients and families of patients undergoing diagnostic tests or procedures, and providing pretest, intratest, and post-test information and support
- Maintaining quality control to prevent or eliminate problems that may interfere with the accuracy and reliability of test results
- Providing education and emotional support at the point of care
- Ensuring completion of testing in a timely and accurate manner
- Collaborating with other health-care professionals in interpreting findings as they relate to planning and implementing total patient care
- Communicating significant alterations in test outcomes to appropriate health-care team members
- Coordinating interdisciplinary efforts

Whether the nurse's role at each level is direct or indirect, the underlying responsibility to the patient, family, and community remains the same.

This book is a reference for nurses, nursing students, and other health-care professionals. It is useful as a clinical tool as well as a supportive text to supplement clinical courses. It guides the nurse in planning what needs to be assessed, monitored, treated, and taught regarding pretest requirements, intratest procedures, and post-test care. It can be used by nursing students at all levels as a textbook in theory classes, integrating laboratory and diagnostic data as one aspect of nursing care; by practicing nurses to update information; and in clinical settings as a quick reference. Designed for use in academic and clinical settings, *Davis's Comprehensive Handbook of Laboratory and Diagnostic Tests—With Nursing Implications* provides a comprehensive reference that allows easy access to information about laboratory and diagnostic tests and procedures. A general overview of how all the tests and procedures included in this book relate to body systems can be found in tables at the end of the monographs. The tests and procedures are presented in this book in alphabetical order by their complete name, allowing the user to locate information quickly without having to first place tests in a specific category or body system. Each monograph is presented in a consistent format for easy identification of specific information at a glance. The following information is provided for each laboratory and diagnostic test:

- Each monograph is titled by the *test name,* given in its commonly used designation, and all monographs in the book are organized in alphabetical order.
- *Synonyms and Acronyms* for each test are listed where appropriate.
- The *Common Use* section includes a brief description of the purpose for the study.
- The *Specimen* section includes the type of specimen usually collected and, where appropriate, the type of collection tube or container commonly recommended. The amount of specimen collected for blood studies reflects the amount of serum, plasma, or whole blood required to perform the test and thus provides a way to project the total number of specimen containers required, because patients usually have multiple laboratory tests requested for a single draw. Specimen requirements vary by laboratory. The amount of specimen collected is usually more than what is minimally required so that additional specimen is available, if needed, for repeat testing (quality-control failure, dilutions, or confirmation of unexpected results). In the case of diagnostic tests, the *type* of procedure (e.g., nuclear medicine, x-ray) is given.
- *Normal Findings* for each monograph include age-specific, gender-specific, and ethnicity-specific variations, when indicated. It is important to consider the normal variation of laboratory values over the life span and across cultures; sometimes what might be considered an abnormal value in one circumstance is actually what is expected in another. Normal findings for laboratory tests are given in conventional and standard international (SI) units. The factor used to convert conventional to SI units is also given. Because laboratory values can vary by method, each laboratory reference range is listed along with the associated methodology.
- The *Description* section includes the study's purpose and insight into how and why the test results can affect health.
- *Indications* are a list of what the test is used for in terms of assessment, evaluation, monitoring, screening, identifying, or assisting in the diagnosis of a clinical condition.
- The *Potential Diagnosis* section presents a list of conditions in which values may be increased or decreased and, in some cases, an explanation of variations that may be encountered.
- *Critical Findings* that may be life threatening or for which particular concern may be indicated are given in conventional and SI units, along with age span considerations where applicable. This section also includes signs and symptoms associated with a critical value as well as possible nursing interventions and the nurse's role in communication of critical findings to the appropriate health-care provider.
- *Interfering Factors* are substances or circumstances that may influence the results of the test, rendering the results invalid or unreliable. Knowledge of interfering factors is an important aspect of quality assurance and includes pharmaceuticals, foods, natural and additive therapies, timing of test in relation to other tests or procedures, collection site, handling of specimen, and underlying patient conditions.
- The *Pretest* section addresses the need to:
  - Positively identify the patient using at least two unique identifiers before providing care, treatment, or services.
  - Provide an explanation to the patient, in the simplest terms possible, of the purpose of the study.

- Obtain pertinent clinical, laboratory, dietary, and therapeutic history of the patient, especially as it pertains to comparison of previous test results, preparation for the test, and identification of potentially interfering factors.
- Explain the requirements and restrictions related to the procedure as well as what to expect; provide the education necessary for the patient to be properly informed.
- Anticipate and allay patient and family concerns or anxieties with consideration of social and cultural issues during interactions.
- Provide for patient safety.
- The *Intratest* section can be used in a quality-control assessment or as a guide to the nurse who may be called on to participate in specimen collection or perform preparatory procedures. It provides:
  - Specific directions for specimen collection and test performance
  - Important information such as patient sensation and expected duration of the procedure
  - Precautions to be taken by the nurse and patient
- The *Post-Test* section provides guidelines regarding:
  - Specific monitoring and therapeutic measures that should be performed after the procedure (e.g., maintaining bedrest, obtaining vital signs to compare with baseline values, signs and symptoms of complications)
  - Specific instructions for the patient and family, such as when to resume usual diet, medications, and activity
  - General nutritional guidelines related to excess or deficit as well as common food sources for dietary replacement
  - Indications for interventions from public health representatives or for special counseling related to test outcomes
  - Indications for follow-up testing that may be required within specific time frames
  - An alphabetical listing of related laboratory and/or diagnostic tests that is intended to provoke a deeper and broader investigation of multiple pieces of information; the tests provide data that, when combined, can form a more complete picture of health or illness
  - Reference to the specific body system tables of related laboratory and diagnostic tests that might bear on a patient's situation

Color and icons are used to facilitate locating critical information at a glance. On the inside front and back covers is a full-color chart describing tube tops used for various blood tests and their recommended order of draw.

Wherever possible, in each monograph, information has been organized alphabetically to make it easier for the reader to quickly locate needed information, as seen in the Indications, Potential Diagnosis, and Interfering Factors (drug lists) sections.

The nursing process is evident throughout the laboratory and diagnostic monographs. Within each phase of the testing procedure, the nurse has certain roles and responsibilities. These should be evident in reading each monograph.

Information provided in the back matter and appendices includes a series of system tables that alphabetically organize laboratory and diagnostic tests by related body systems; a summary of guidelines for patient preparation with specimen collection procedures and materials; a summary of common potential nursing diagnoses associated with laboratory and diagnostic testing; a summary chart that details age-specific nursing care guidelines with suggested approaches to persons at various developmental stages to assist the provider in facilitating cooperation and understanding; a summary chart of transfusion reactions, their signs and symptoms, associated laboratory findings, and potential nursing interventions; an introduction to CLIA (Clinical Laboratory Improvement Amendments) with an explanation of the different levels of testing complexity; a list of some of the herbs and nutraceuticals associated with adverse clinical reactions or drug interactions related to the affected body system; and guidelines for standard precautions.

The index has been enhanced to include the addition of new tests, conditions, and other key words.

This book is also about teaching. The newly revised Instructor Guide and Student Guide have been updated with broadened age-related categories designed to enhance clinical communication. Chapter content in the guides is coordinated, making them much easier to use in the classroom setting. The newly added online Case Studies are written in a format to help the novice learn how to clinically reason by using nursing process to problem solve. Cases are purposefully designed to promote discussion of situations that may occur in the clinical setting. Situations may be medical, ethical, family related, patient related, nurse related and any combination in between. Additional educationally supportive materials are provided for the instructor and student in an *Instructor's Guide*, available on the Instructor's Resource Disk (CD) and posted at DavisPlus (http://davisplus.fadavis.com). Organized by nursing curriculum, presentations and case studies with emphasis on laboratory and diagnostic test–related information and nursing implications have been developed for selected conditions and body systems, including sensory, obstetric, and nutrition coverage. Open-ended and NCLEX-type multiple-choice questions as well as suggested critical-thinking activities are provided. This supplemental material aids the instructor in integrating laboratory and diagnostic materials in assessment and clinical courses and provides examples of activities to enhance student learning.

Newly developed case studies for this fifth edition have been added to a robust collection of online material for students and educators posted at the DavisPlus Web site (http://davisplus.fadavis.com):

- A searchable library of mini-monographs for all the active tests included in the text. The mini-monograph gives each test's full name, synonyms and acronyms, specimen type (laboratory tests) or area of application (diagnostic tests), reference ranges or contrast, and results.
- An archive of full monographs of retired tests that are referenced by mini-monographs in the text.
- Interactive drag-and-drop, quiz-show, flash card, and multiple-choice exercises.
- A printable file of critical findings for laboratory and diagnostic tests.
- All the instructor and student material from the Instructor's Resource Disk.
- Case studies with both an instructor and student version for assistance with clinical development in the practice setting.
- PowerPoint presentation of laboratory and diagnostic pretest, intratest, and post-test concepts integrated with nursing process.

The authors hope that the changes and additions made to the book and its CD and Web-based ancillaries will reward users with an expanded understanding of and appreciation for the place laboratory and diagnostic testing holds in the provision of high-quality nursing care and will make it easy for instructors to integrate this important content in their curricula.

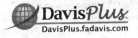

DavisPlus.fadavis.com

Laboratory and diagnostic testing. The words themselves often conjure up cold and impersonal images of needles, specimens lined up in collection containers, and high-tech electronic equipment. But they do not stand alone. They are tied to, bound with, and tell of health or disease in the blood and tissue of a person. Laboratory and diagnostic studies augment the health-care provider's assessment of the quality of an individual's physical being. Test results guide the plans and interventions geared toward strengthening life's quality and endurance. Beyond the pounding noise of the MRI, the cold steel of the x-ray table, the sting of the needle, the invasive collection of fluids and tissue, and the probing and inspection is the gathering of evidence that supports the health-care provider's ability to discern the course of a disease and the progression of its treatment. Laboratory and diagnostic data must be viewed with thought and compassion, however, as well as with microscopes and machines. We must remember that behind the specimen and test result is the person from whom it came, a person who is someone's son, daughter, mother, father, husband, wife, friend.

This book is written to help health-care providers in their understanding and interpretation of laboratory and diagnostic procedures and their outcomes. Just as important, it is dedicated to all health-care professionals who experience the wonders in the science of laboratory and diagnostic testing, performed and interpreted in a caring and efficient manner.

Reviewers

Nell Britton, MSN, RN, CNE
Nursing Faculty
Trident Technical College Nursing
    Division
Charleston, South Carolina

Cheryl Cassis, MSN, RN
Professor of Nursing
Belmont Technical College
St. Clairsville, Ohio

Pamela Ellis, RN, MSHCA, MSN
Nursing Faculty
Mohave Community College
Bullhead City, Arizona

Stephanie Franks, MSN, RN
Professor of Nursing
St. Louis Community College-Meramec
St. Louis, Missouri

Linda Lott, MSN
AD Nursing Instructor
Itawamba Community College
Fulton, Mississippi

Martha Olson, RN, BSN, MS
Nursing Associate Professor
Iowa Lakes Community College
Emmetsburg, Iowa

Barbara Thompson, RN, BScN,
    MScN
Professor of Nursing
Sault College
Sault Ste. Marie, Ontario

Edward C. Walton, MS, APN-C, NP-C
Assistant Professor of Nursing
Richard Stockton College
    of New Jersey
Galloway, New Jersey

Jean Ann Wilson, RN, BSN
Coordinator Norton Annex
Colby Community College
Norton, Kansas

Contents

Acetylcholine Receptor Antibody

SYNONYM/ACRONYM: AChR (AChR-binding antibody, AChR-blocking antibody, and AChR-modulating antibody).

COMMON USE: To assist in confirming the diagnosis of myasthenia gravis (MG).

SPECIMEN: Serum (1 mL) collected in a red-top tube.

NORMAL FINDINGS: (Method: Radioimmunoassay) AChR binding antibody: Less than 0.4 nmol/L, AChR blocking antibody: Less than 15% blocking, and AChR modulating antibody: Less than 20% modulating.

DESCRIPTION: Normally when impulses travel down a nerve, the nerve ending releases a neurotransmitter called acetylcholine (ACh), which binds to receptor sites in the neuromuscular junction, eventually resulting in muscle contraction. Once the neuromuscular junction is polarized, ACh is rapidly metabolized by the enzyme acetylcholinesterase. When present, AChR-binding antibodies can activate complement and create a complex of ACh, AChR-binding antibodies, and complement. This complex renders ACh unavailable for muscle receptor sites. If AChR binding antibodies are not detected, and MG is strongly suspected, AChR-blocking and AChR-modulating antibodies may be ordered. AChR-blocking antibodies impair or prevent ACh from attaching to receptor sites on the muscle membrane, resulting in poor muscle contraction. AChR-modulating antibodies destroy AChR sites, interfering with neuromuscular transmission. The lack of ACh bound to muscle receptor sites results in muscle weakness. Antibodies to AChR sites are present in 90% of patients with generalized MG and in 55% to 70% of patients who either have ocular forms of MG or are in remission. Approximately 10% to 15% of people with confirmed MG do not demonstrate detectable levels of AChR-binding, -blocking, or -modulating antibodies. MG is an acquired autoimmune disorder that can occur at any age. Its exact cause is unknown, and it seems to strike women between the ages of 20 and 40 years; men appear to be affected later in life than women. It can affect any voluntary muscle, but muscles that control eye, eyelid, facial movement, and swallowing are most frequently affected. Antibodies may not be detected in the first 6 to 12 months after the first appearance of symptoms. MG is a common complication associated with thymoma. The relationship between the thymus gland and MG is not completely understood. It is believed that miscommunication in the thymus gland directed at developing immune cells may trigger the development of autoantibodies responsible for MG. Remission after thymectomy is associated with a progressive decrease in antibody level. Other markers used in the study of MG include striational muscle antibodies, thyroglobulin, HLA-B8, and HLA-DR3. These antibodies are often undetectable in the early stages of MG.

INDICATIONS
- Confirm the presence but not the severity of MG
- Detect subclinical MG in the presence of thymoma

A

- Monitor the effectiveness of immunosuppressive therapy for MG
- Monitor the remission stage of MG

POTENTIAL DIAGNOSIS

Increased in
- Autoimmune liver disease
- Generalized MG *(Defective transmission of nerve impulses to muscles evidenced by muscle weakness. It occurs when normal communication between the nerve and muscle is interrupted at the neuromuscular junction. It is believed that miscommunication in the thymus gland directed at developing immune cells may trigger the development of autoantibodies responsible for MG.)*
- Lambert-Eaton myasthenic syndrome
- Primary lung cancer
- Thymoma associated with MG *(Defective transmission of nerve impulses to muscles evidenced by muscle weakness. It occurs when normal communication between the nerve and muscle is interrupted at the neuromuscular junction. It is believed that miscommunication in the thymus gland directed at developing immune cells may trigger the development of autoantibodies responsible for MG.)*

Decreased in
- Post-thymectomy *(The thymus gland produces the T lymphocytes responsible for cell-mediated immunity. T cells also help control B-cell development for the production of antibodies. T-cell response is directed at cells in the body that have been infected by bacteria, viruses, parasites, fungi, or protozoans. T cells also provide immune surveillance for cancerous cells. Removal of the thymus gland is strongly associated with a decrease in AChR antibody levels.)*

CRITICAL FINDINGS: N/A

INTERFERING FACTORS
- Drugs that may increase AChR levels include penicillamine (long-term use may cause a reversible syndrome that produces clinical, serological, and electrophysiological findings indistinguishable from MG).
- Biological false-positive results may be associated with amyotrophic lateral sclerosis, autoimmune hepatitis, Lambert-Eaton myasthenic syndrome, primary biliary cirrhosis, and encephalomyeloneuropathies associated with carcinoma of the lung.
- Immunosuppressive therapy is the recommended treatment for MG; prior immunosuppressive drug administration may result in negative test results.
- Recent radioactive scans or radiation within 1 wk of the test can interfere with test results when radioimmunoassay is the test method.

NURSING IMPLICATIONS AND PROCEDURE

PRETEST:
- Positively identify the patient using at least two unique identifiers before providing care, treatment, or services.
- *Patient Teaching:* Inform the patient that the test is used to identify antibodies responsible for decreased neuromuscular transmission and associated muscle weakness.
- Obtain a history of the patient's complaints, including a list of known allergens, especially allergies or sensitivities to latex, and any prior complications with general anesthesia.
- Obtain a history of the patient's musculoskeletal system, symptoms, and results of previously performed laboratory tests and diagnostic and surgical procedures.

- Note any recent procedures that can interfere with test results.
- Obtain a list of the patient's current medications, including herbs, nutritional supplements, and nutraceuticals (see Appendix F).
- Review the procedure with the patient. Inform the patient that specimen collection takes approximately 5 to 10 min. Address concerns about pain and explain that there may be some discomfort during the venipuncture.
- *Sensitivity to social and cultural issues,* as well as concern for modesty, is important in providing psychological support before, during, and after the procedure. There are no food, fluid, or medication restrictions unless by medical direction.

INTRATEST:

- If the patient has a history of allergic reaction to latex, avoid the use of equipment containing latex.
- Instruct the patient to cooperate fully and to follow directions. Direct the patient to breathe normally and to avoid unnecessary movement.
- Observe standard precautions, and follow the general guidelines in Appendix A. Positively identify the patient, and label the appropriate specimen container with the corresponding patient demographics, initials of the person collecting the specimen, date, and time of collection. Perform a venipuncture.
- Remove the needle and apply direct pressure with dry gauze to stop bleeding. Observe/assess venipuncture site for bleeding or hematoma formation and secure gauze with adhesive bandage.
- Promptly transport the specimen to the laboratory for processing and analysis.

POST-TEST:

- A report of the results will be made available to the requesting health-care provider (HCP), who will discuss the results with the patient.
- Recognize anxiety related to test results, and be supportive of activity challenges related to lack of neuromuscular control, anticipated loss of independence and fear of death. Discuss the implications of positive test results on the patient's lifestyle. It is important to note that a

diagnosis of MG should be based on abnormal findings from two different diagnostic tests. These tests include AChR antibody assay, edrophonium test, repetitive nerve stimulation, and single-fiber electromyography. Thyrotoxicosis may occur in conjunction with MG; related thyroid testing may be indicated. MG patients may also produce antibodies that demonstrate reactivity in tests like Antinuclear antibody and Rheumatoid factor that are not primarily associated with MG.
- Evaluate test results in relation to future general anesthesia, especially regarding therapeutic management of MG with cholinesterase inhibitors. Succinylcholine-sensitive patients may be unable to metabolize the anesthetic quickly, resulting in prolonged or unrecoverable apnea.
- Provide teaching and information regarding the clinical implications of the test results as appropriate.
- Educate the patient regarding access to counseling services. Provide contact information, if desired, for the Myasthenia Gravis Foundation of America (www.myasthenia.org) and the Muscular Dystrophy Association (www.mdausa.org).
- Reinforce information given by the patient's HCP regarding further testing, treatment, or referral to another HCP. Answer any questions or address any concerns voiced by the patient or family.
- Depending on the results of this procedure, additional testing may be performed to evaluate or monitor progression of the disease process and determine the need for a change in therapy. If a diagnosis of MG is made, a computed tomography (CT) scan of the chest should be performed to rule out thymoma. Evaluate test results in relation to the patient's symptoms and other tests performed.

RELATED MONOGRAPHS:

- Related tests include ANA, antithyroglobulin and antithyroid peroxidase antibodies, CT chest, myoglobin, pseudocholinesterase, RF, TSH, and total T_4.
- Refer to the Musculoskeletal System table at the end of the book for related tests by body system.

A

Acid Phosphatase, Prostatic

SYNONYM/ACRONYM: Prostatic acid phosphatase, *o*-phosphoric monoester phosphohydrolase, AcP PAP

COMMON USE: To assist in staging prostate cancer and document evidence of sexual intercourse through semen identification in alleged cases of rape and sexual abuse.

SPECIMEN: Serum (1 mL) collected in a red-top tube.
A swab with vaginal secretions may be submitted in the appropriate transfer container. Other material such as clothing may be submitted for analysis. Consult the laboratory or emergency services department for the proper specimen collection instructions and containers.

NORMAL FINDINGS: (Method: Immunochemiluminometric)

Conventional & SI Units
Less than 3.5 ng/mL

Values are elevated at birth, decrease by 6 mo, increase at approximately 10 yr through puberty, level off through adulthood, and may increase in advancing age.

POTENTIAL DIAGNOSIS

Increased in

AcP is released from any damaged cell in which it is stored, so diseases of the bone, prostate, and liver that cause cellular destruction demonstrate elevated AcP levels. Conditions that result in abnormal elevations of cells that contain AcP (e.g., leukemia, thrombocytosis) or conditions that result in rapid cellular destruction (sickle cell crisis) also reflect increased levels.

- Acute myelogenous leukemia
- After prostate surgery or biopsy
- Benign prostatic hypertrophy
- Liver disease
- Lysosomal storage diseases (Gaucher's disease and Niemann-Pick disease) *(AcP is stored in the lysosomes of blood cells, and increased levels are present in lysosomal storage diseases)*
- Metastatic bone cancer
- Paget's disease
- Prostatic cancer
- Prostatic infarct
- Prostatitis
- Sickle cell crisis
- Thrombocytosis

Decreased in: N/A

CRITICAL FINDINGS: N/A

Find and print out the full monograph at DavisPlus (http://davisplus.fadavis .com, keyword Van Leeuwen).

Adrenal Gland Scan

SYNONYM/ACRONYM: Adrenal scintiscan.

COMMON USE: To assist in the diagnosis of Cushing's syndrome and differentiate between adrenal gland cancer and infection.

AREA OF APPLICATION: Adrenal gland.

CONTRAST: Intravenous radioactive NP-59 (iodomethyl-19-norcholesterol) or metaiodobenzylguanidine (MIBG).

DESCRIPTION: This nuclear medicine study evaluates function of the adrenal glands. The secretory function of the adrenal glands is controlled primarily by the anterior pituitary, which produces adrenocorticotropic hormone (ACTH). ACTH stimulates the adrenal cortex to produce cortisone and secrete aldosterone. Adrenal imaging is most useful in differentiation of hyperplasia from adenoma in primary aldosteronism when computed tomography (CT) and magnetic resonance imaging (MRI) findings are equivocal. High concentrations of cholesterol (the precursor in the synthesis of adrenocorticosteroids, including aldosterone) are stored in the adrenal cortex. This allows the radionuclide, which attaches to the cholesterol, to be used in identifying pathology in the secretory function of the adrenal cortex. The uptake of the radionuclide occurs gradually over time; imaging is performed within 24 to 48 hr of injection of the radionuclide dose and continued daily for 3 to 5 days. Imaging reveals increased uptake, unilateral or bilateral uptake, or absence of uptake in the detection of pathological processes.

Following prescanning treatment with corticosteroids, suppression studies can be done to differentiate the presence of tumor from hyperplasia of the glands.

INDICATIONS
- Aid in the diagnosis of Cushing's syndrome and aldosteronism
- Aid in the diagnosis of gland tissue destruction caused by infection, infarction, neoplasm, or suppression
- Aid in locating adrenergic tumors
- Determine adrenal suppressibility with prescan administration of corticosteroid to diagnose and localize adrenal adenoma, aldosteronomas, androgen excess, and low-renin hypertension
- Differentiate between asymmetric hyperplasia and asymmetry from aldosteronism with dexamethasone suppression test

POTENTIAL DIAGNOSIS

Normal findings in
- No evidence of tumors, infection, infarction, or suppression
- Normal bilateral uptake of radionuclide and secretory function of adrenal cortex
- Normal salivary glands and urinary bladder; vague shape of the liver and spleen sometimes seen

A

Abnormal findings in
- Adrenal gland suppression
- Adrenal infarction
- Adrenal tumor
- Hyperplasia
- Infection
- Pheochromocytoma

CRITICAL FINDINGS: N/A

INTERFERING FACTORS

This procedure is contraindicated for
- Patients who are pregnant or suspected of being pregnant unless the potential benefits of the procedure far outweigh the risks to the fetus and mother.

Factors that may impair clear imaging
- Retained barium from a previous radiological procedure.
- Inability of the patient to cooperate or remain still during the procedure because of age, significant pain, or mental status.

Other considerations
- Improper injection of the radionuclide may allow the tracer to seep deep into the muscle tissue, producing erroneous hot spots.
- Consultation with a health-care provider (HCP) should occur before the procedure for radiation safety concerns regarding younger patients or patients who are lactating.
- Risks associated with radiation overexposure can result from frequent x-ray or radionuclide procedures. Personnel working in the examination area should wear badges to record their radiation exposure level.

NURSING IMPLICATIONS AND PROCEDURE

PRETEST:

▶ Positively identify the patient using at least two unique identifiers before providing care, treatment, or services.

Patient Teaching: Inform the patient this procedure can visualize and assess the function of the adrenal gland, which is located near the kidney.

▶ Obtain a history of the patient's complaints, including a list of known allergens.

▶ Obtain a history of the patient's endocrine system, symptoms, and results of previously performed laboratory tests and diagnostic and surgical procedures.

▶ All adrenal blood tests should be done before doing this test.

▶ Record the date of last menstrual period and determine the possibility of pregnancy in perimenopausal women.

▶ Obtain a list of the patient's current medications, including herbs, nutritional supplements, and nutraceuticals (see Appendix F).

▶ Review the procedure with the patient. Address concerns about pain and explain that there may be moments of discomfort and some pain experienced during the test. Inform the patient that the procedure is usually performed in a nuclear medicine department by a nuclear medicine technologist with support staff, and it takes approximately 1 to 2 hr each day. Inform the patient the test usually involves a prolonged scanning schedule over a period of days.

▶ Administer saturated solution of potassium iodide (SSKI) 24 hr before the study to prevent thyroid uptake of the free radioactive iodine.

▶ *Sensitivity to social and cultural issues,* as well as concern for modesty, is important in providing psychological support before, during, and after the procedure.

▶ Explain that an IV line may be inserted to allow infusion of radionuclides or IV fluids.

▶ There are no food, fluid, or medication restrictions unless by medical direction.

▶ Instruct the patient to remove jewelry and other metallic objects from the area to be examined.

▶ *Make sure a written and informed consent has been signed prior to the procedure and before administering any medications.*

INTRATEST:

- Observe standard precautions, and follow the general guidelines in Appendix A. Positively identify the patient.
- Ensure that the patient has removed external metallic objects from the area to be examined prior to the procedure.
- Have emergency equipment readily available.
- Instruct the patient to void prior to the procedure and to change into the gown, robe, and foot coverings provided.
- Insert an IV line, and inject the radionuclide IV on day 1; images are taken on days 1, 2, and 3. Imaging is done from the urinary bladder to the base of the skull to scan for a primary tumor. Each image takes 20 min, and total imaging time is 1 to 2 hr per day.
- Instruct the patient to cooperate fully and to follow directions. Instruct the patient to remain still throughout the procedure because movement produces unreliable results.

POST-TEST:

- A report of the results will be made available to the requesting HCP, who will discuss the results with the patient.
- Unless contraindicated, advise the patient to drink increased amounts of fluids for 24 to 48 hrs to eliminate the radionuclide from the body. Inform the patient that radionuclide is eliminated from the body within 24 to 48 hr.
- No other radionuclide tests should be scheduled for 24 to 48 hr after this procedure.
- Observe/assess the needle site for bleeding, hematoma formation, and inflammation.
- Instruct the patient in the care and assessment of the injection site.
- Instruct the patient to apply cold compresses to the puncture site as needed to reduce discomfort or edema.
- If a woman who is breastfeeding must have a nuclear scan, she should not breastfeed the infant until the radionuclide has been eliminated. This could take as long as 3 days. Instruct her to express the milk and discard it during the 3-day period to prevent cessation of milk production.
- Instruct the patient to immediately flush the toilet and to meticulously wash hands with soap and water after each voiding for 48 hrs after the procedure.
- Instruct all caregivers to wear gloves when discarding urine for 48 hrs after the procedure. Wash gloved hands with soap and water before removing gloves. Then wash ungloved hands after the gloves are removed.
- Recognize anxiety related to test results. Discuss the implications of abnormal test results on the patient's lifestyle. Provide teaching and information regarding the clinical implications of the test results, as appropriate.
- Reinforce information given by the patient's HCP regarding further testing, treatment, or referral to another HCP. Advise the patient that SSKI (120 mg/day) will be administered for 10 days after the injection of the radionuclide. Answer any questions or address any concerns voiced by the patient or family.
- Depending on the results of this procedure, additional testing may be needed to evaluate or monitor progression of the disease process and determine the need for a change in therapy. Evaluate test results in relation to the patient's symptoms and other tests performed.

RELATED MONOGRAPHS:

- Related tests include ACTH and challenge tests, aldosterone, angiography adrenal, catecholamines, CT abdomen, cortisol and challenge tests, HVA, MRI abdomen, metanephrines, potassium, renin, sodium, and VMA.
- Refer to the Endocrine System table at the end of the book for related tests by body system.

A

Adrenocorticotropic Hormone (and Challenge Tests)

SYNONYM/ACRONYM: Corticotropin, ACTH.

COMMON USE: To assist in the investigation of adrenocortical dysfunction using ACTH and cortisol levels in diagnosing disorders such as Addison's disease, Cushing's disease, and Cushing's syndrome.

SPECIMEN: Plasma (2 mL) from a lavender-top (EDTA) tube for adrenocorticotropic hormone (ACTH) and serum (1 mL) from a red-top tube for cortisol and 11-deoxycortisol. Collect specimens in a prechilled heparinized plastic syringe, and carefully transfer into collection containers by gentle injection to avoid hemolysis. Alternatively, specimens can be collected in prechilled lavender- and red-top tubes. Tiger- and green-top (heparin) tubes are also acceptable for cortisol, but take care to use the same type of collection container for serial measurements. Immediately transport specimen, tightly capped and in an ice slurry, to the laboratory. The specimens should be immediately processed. Plasma for ACTH analysis should be transferred to a plastic container.

Procedure	Medication Administered, Adult Dosage	Recommended Collection Times
ACTH stimulation, rapid test	1 mcg (low-dose protocol) cosyntropin IM	Three cortisol levels: baseline immediately before bolus, 30 min after bolus, and 60 min after bolus
Corticotropin-releasing hormone (CRH) stimulation	IV dose of 1 mcg/kg human CRH	Eight cortisol and eight ACTH levels: baseline collected 15 min before injection, 0 min before injection, and then 5, 15, 30, 60, 120, and 180 min after injection
Dexamethasone suppression (overnight)	Oral dose of 1 mg dexamethasone (Decadron) at 11 p.m.	Collect cortisol at 8 a.m. on the morning after the dexamethasone dose
Metyrapone stimulation (overnight)	Oral dose of 30 mg/kg metyrapone with snack at midnight	Collect cortisol, 11-deoxycortisol, and ACTH at 8 a.m. on the morning after the metyrapone dose

IM = intramuscular, IV = intravenous.

NORMAL FINDINGS: (Method: Immunochemiluminescent assay for ACTH and cortisol; HPLC/MS-MS for 11-deoxycortisol)

ACTH

Age	Conventional Units	SI Units (Conventional Units × 0.22)
Cord blood	50–570 pg/mL	11–125 pmol/L
Newborn	10–185 pg/mL	2–41 pmol/L
1 wk-9 yr	5–46 pg/mL	1.1–10.1 pmol/L
10–18 yr	6–55 pg/mL	1.3–12.1 pmol/L
19 yr-Adult		
Male supine (specimen collected in morning)	7–69 pg/mL	1.5–15.2 pmol/L
Female supine (specimen collected in morning)	6–58 pg/mL	1.3–12.8 pmol/L

Values may be unchanged or slightly elevated in healthy older adults. Long-term use of corticosteroids, to treat arthritis and autoimmune diseases, may suppress secretion of ACTH.

ACTH Challenge Tests

ACTH (Cosyntropin) Stimulated, Rapid Test	Conventional Units	SI Units (Conventional Units × 27.6)
Baseline	Cortisol greater than 5 mcg/dL	Greater than 138 nmol/L
30- or 60-min response	Cortisol 18–20 mcg/dL or incremental increase of 7 mcg/dL over baseline value	497–552 nmol/L

Corticotropin-Releasing Hormone Stimulated	Conventional Units	SI Units (Conventional Units × 27.6)
	Cortisol peaks at greater than 20 mcg/dL within 30–60 min	Greater than 552 nmol/L
		SI Units (Conventional Units × 0.22)
	ACTH increases twofold to fourfold within 30–60 min	Twofold to fourfold increase within 30–60 min

A

Dexamethasone Suppressed Overnight Test	Conventional Units	SI Units (Conventional Units × 27.6)
	Cortisol less than 1.8 mcg/dL next day	Less than 49.7 nmol/L

Metyrapone Stimulated Overnight Test	Conventional Units	SI Units (Conventional Units × 27.6)
	Cortisol less than 3 mcg/dL next day	Less than 83 nmol/L
		SI Units (Conventional Units × 0.22)
	ACTH greater than 75 pg/mL	Greater than 16.5 pmol/L
		SI Units (Conventional Units × 28.9)
	11-deoxycortisol greater than 7 mcg/dL	Greater than 202 nmol/L

DESCRIPTION: Hypothalamic-releasing factor stimulates the release of ACTH from the anterior pituitary gland. ACTH stimulates adrenal cortex secretion of glucocorticoids, androgens, and, to a lesser degree, mineralocorticoids. Cortisol is the major glucocorticoid secreted by the adrenal cortex. ACTH and cortisol test results are evaluated together because a change in one normally causes a change in the other. ACTH secretion is stimulated by insulin, metyrapone, and vasopressin. It is decreased by dexamethasone. Cortisol excess from any source is termed *Cushing's syndrome*. Cortisol excess resulting from ACTH excess produced by the pituitary is termed *Cushing's disease*. ACTH levels exhibit a diurnal variation, peaking between 6 and 8 a.m. and reaching the lowest point between 6 and 11 p.m. Evening levels are generally one-half to two-thirds lower than morning levels. Cortisol levels also vary diurnally, with the peak values occurring during the morning and lowest levels occurring in the evening.

INDICATIONS
• Determine adequacy of replacement therapy in congenital adrenal hyperplasia
• Determine adrenocortical dysfunction
• Differentiate between increased ACTH release with decreased cortisol levels and decreased ACTH release with increased cortisol levels

POTENTIAL DIAGNOSIS

ACTH Result
Because ACTH and cortisol secretion exhibit diurnal variation with

values being highest in the morning, a lack of change in values from morning to evening is clinically significant. Decreased concentrations of hormones secreted by the pituitary gland and its target organs are observed in hypopituitarism. In primary adrenal insufficiency (Addison's disease), because of adrenal gland destruction by tumor, infectious process, or immune reaction, ACTH levels are elevated while cortisol levels are decreased. Both ACTH and cortisol levels are decreased in secondary adrenal insufficiency (i.e., secondary to pituitary insufficiency). Excess ACTH can be produced ectopically by various lung cancers such as oat-cell carcinoma and large-cell carcinoma of the lung and by benign bronchial carcinoid tumor.

Challenge Tests and Results

The ACTH (cosyntropin) stimulated rapid test directly evaluates adrenal gland function and indirectly evaluates pituitary gland and hypothalamus function. Cosyntropin is a synthetic form of ACTH. A baseline cortisol level is collected before the injection of cosyntropin. Specimens are subsequently collected at 30- and 60-min intervals. If the adrenal glands function normally, cortisol levels rise significantly after administration of cosyntropin.

The CRH stimulation test works as well as the dexamethasone suppression test (DST) in distinguishing Cushing's disease from conditions in which ACTH is secreted ectopically (e.g., tumors not located in the pituitary gland that secrete ACTH). Patients with pituitary tumors tend to respond to CRH stimulation, whereas those with ectopic tumors do not. Patients with adrenal insufficiency demonstrate one of

three patterns depending on the underlying cause:

* Primary adrenal insufficiency— high baseline ACTH (in response to IV-administered ACTH) and low cortisol levels pre- and post-IV ACTH.
* Secondary adrenal insufficiency (pituitary)—low baseline ACTH that does not respond to ACTH stimulation. Cortisol levels do not increase after stimulation.
* Tertiary adrenal insufficiency (hypothalamic)—low baseline ACTH with an exaggerated and prolonged response to stimulation. Cortisol levels usually do not reach 20 mcg/dL.

The DST is useful in differentiating the causes of increased cortisol levels. Dexamethasone is a synthetic glucocorticoid that is significantly more potent than cortisol. It works by negative feedback. It suppresses the release of ACTH in patients with a normal hypothalamus. A cortisol level less than 1.8 mcg/dL usually excludes Cushing's syndrome. With the DST, a baseline morning cortisol level is collected, and the patient is given a 1-mg dose of dexamethasone at bedtime. A second specimen is collected the following morning. If cortisol levels have not been suppressed, adrenal adenoma is suspected. The DST also produces abnormal results in the presence of certain psychiatric illnesses (e.g., endogenous depression).

The metyrapone stimulation test is used to distinguish corticotropin-dependent causes (pituitary Cushing's disease and ectopic Cushing's disease) from corticotropin-independent causes (e.g., carcinoma of the lung or thyroid) of increased cortisol levels. Metyrapone inhibits the conversion of 11-deoxycortisol to

A

cortisol. Cortisol levels should decrease to less than 3 mcg/dL if normal pituitary stimulation by ACTH occurs after an oral dose of metyrapone. Specimen collection and administration of the medication are performed as with the overnight dexamethasone test.

Increased in
Overproduction of ACTH can occur as a direct result of either disease (e.g., primary or ectopic tumor that secretes ACTH) or stimulation by physical or emotional stress, or it can be an indirect response to abnormalities in the complex feedback mechanisms involving the pituitary gland, hypothalamus, or adrenal glands.

ACTH Increased In
- Addison's disease *(primary adrenocortical hypofunction)*
- Carcinoid syndrome
- Congenital adrenal hyperplasia
- Cushing's disease *(pituitary-dependent adrenal hyperplasia)*
- Depression
- Ectopic ACTH-producing tumors
- Menstruation
- Nelson's syndrome *(ACTH-producing pituitary tumors)*
- Non-insulin-dependent diabetes
- Pregnancy
- Sepsis
- Septic shock

Decreased in
Secondary adrenal insufficiency due to hypopituitarism (inadequate production by the pituitary) can result in decreased levels of ACTH. Conditions that result in overproduction or availability of high levels of cortisol can also result in decreased levels of ACTH.

ACTH Decreased in
- Adrenal adenoma
- Adrenal cancer

- Cushing's syndrome
- Exogenous steroid therapy

CRITICAL FINDINGS: N/A

INTERFERING FACTORS
- Drugs that may increase ACTH levels include insulin, metoclopramide, metyrapone, mifepristone (RU 486), and vasopressin.
- Drugs that may decrease ACTH levels include corticosteroids (e.g., dexamethasone) and pravastatin.
- Test results are affected by the time the test is done because ACTH levels vary diurnally, with the highest values occurring between 6 and 8 a.m. and the lowest values occurring at night. Samples should be collected at the same time of day, between 6 and 8 a.m.
- Excessive physical activity can produce elevated levels.
- ❖ The metyrapone stimulation test is contraindicated in patients with suspected adrenal insufficiency.
- ❖ Metyrapone may cause gastrointestinal distress and/or confusion. Administer oral dose of metyrapone with milk and snack.
- ❖ Rapid clearance of metyrapone, resulting in falsely increased cortisol levels, may occur if the patient is taking drugs that enhance steroid metabolism (e.g., phenytoin, rifampin, phenobarbital, mitotane, and corticosteroids). The requesting health-care provider (HCP) should be consulted prior to a metyrapone stimulation test regarding a decision to withhold these medications

NURSING IMPLICATIONS AND PROCEDURE

PRETEST:

▶ Positively identify the patient using at least two unique identifiers before providing care, treatment, or services.

▶ *Patient Teaching:* Inform the patient this test can assist in evaluating the amount of hormone produced by the pituitary gland located at the base of the brain.

▶ Obtain a history of the patient's complaints, including a list of known allergens, especially allergies or sensitivities to latex.

▶ Obtain a history of the patient's endocrine system, symptoms, and results of previously performed laboratory tests and diagnostic and surgical procedures.

▶ Note any recent procedures that can interfere with test results.

▶ Obtain a list of the patient's current medications, especially drugs that enhance steroid metabolism, including herbs, nutritional supplements, and nutraceuticals (see Appendix F).

▶ Weigh patient and report weight to pharmacy for dosing of metyrapone (30 mg/kg body weight).

▶ Review the procedure with the patient. When ACTH hypersecretion is suspected, a second sample may be requested between 6 and 8 p.m. to determine if changes are the result of diurnal variation in ACTH levels. Inform the patient that more than one sample may be necessary to ensure accurate results, and samples are obtained at specific times to determine high and low levels of ACTH. Inform the patient that each specimen collection takes approximately 5 to 10 min. Address concerns about pain and explain that there may be some discomfort during the venipuncture.

▶ *Sensitivity to social and cultural issues,* as well as concern for modesty, is important in providing psychological support before, during, and after the procedure.

▶ There are no food, fluid, or medication restrictions unless by medical direction.

▶ Drugs that enhance steroid metabolism may be withheld by medical direction prior to metyrapone stimulation testing.

▶ Instruct the patient to refrain from strenuous exercise for 12 hr before the test and to remain in bed or at rest for 1 hr immediately before the test. Avoid smoking and alcohol use.

▶ Prepare an ice slurry in a cup or plastic bag to have on hand for immediate transport of the specimen to the laboratory.

INTRATEST:

▶ Ensure that strenuous exercise was avoided for 12 hr before the test and that 1 hr of bedrest was taken immediately before the test. Samples should be collected between 6 and 8 a.m.

▶ Have emergency equipment readily available in case of adverse reaction to metyrapone.

▶ If the patient has a history of allergic reaction to latex, avoid the use of equipment containing latex.

▶ Instruct the patient to cooperate fully and to follow directions. Direct the patient to breathe normally and to avoid unnecessary movement.

▶ Observe standard precautions, and follow the general guidelines in Appendix A. Positively identify the patient, and label the appropriate tubes with the corresponding patient demographics, date, and time of collection. Perform a venipuncture; collect the specimen in a prechilled plastic heparinized syringe or in prechilled collection containers as listed under the "Specimen" subheading.

▶ Adverse reactions to metyrapone include nausea and vomiting (N/V), abdominal pain, headache, dizziness, sedation, allergic rash, decreased white blood cell (WBC)

A

count, and bone marrow depression. Signs and symptoms of overdose or acute adrenocortical insufficiency include cardiac arrhythmias, hypotension, dehydration, anxiety, confusion, weakness, impairment of consciousness, N/V, epigastric pain, diarrhea, hyponatremia, and hyperkalemia.

▶ Remove the needle and apply direct pressure with dry gauze to stop bleeding. Observe/assess venipuncture site for bleeding or hematoma formation and secure gauze with adhesive bandage.

▶ Promptly transport the specimen to the laboratory for processing and analysis. The tightly capped sample should be placed in an ice slurry immediately after collection. Information on the specimen label should be protected from water in the ice slurry by first placing the specimen in a protective plastic bag.

POST-TEST:

▶ A report of the results will be made available to the requesting HCP, who will discuss the results with the patient.
▶ Instruct the patient to resume normal activity as directed by the HCP.
▶ Recognize anxiety related to test results, and offer support. Provide

contact information, if desired, for the Cushing's Support and Research Foundation (www.csrf.net).
▶ Reinforce information given by the patient's HCP regarding further testing, treatment, or referral to another HCP. Answer any questions or address any concerns voiced by the patient or family.
▶ Depending on the results of this procedure, additional testing may be performed to evaluate or monitor progression of the disease process and determine the need for a change in therapy. If a diagnosis of Cushing's disease is made, pituitary computed tomography (CT) or magnetic resonance imaging (MRI) may be indicated prior to surgery. If a diagnosis of ectopic corticotropin syndrome is made, abdominal CT or MRI may be indicated prior to surgery. Evaluate test results in relation to the patient's symptoms and other tests performed.

RELATED MONOGRAPHS:

▶ Related tests include cortisol and challenge tests, CT abdomen, CT pituitary, MRI abdomen, MRI pituitary, TSH, thyroxine, and US abdomen.
▶ See the Endocrine System table at the end of the book for related tests by body system.

Alanine Aminotransferase

SYNONYM/ACRONYM: Serum glutamic pyruvic transaminase (SGPT), ALT.

COMMON USE: To assess liver function related to liver disease and/or damage.

SPECIMEN: Serum (1 mL) collected in a red- or tiger-top tube. Plasma (1 mL) collected in a green-top (heparin) tube is also acceptable.

NORMAL FINDINGS: (Method: Spectrophotometry)

Age	Conventional & SI Units
Newborn–12 mo	13–45 units/L
13 mo–60 yr	
Male	10–40 units/L
Female	7–35 units/L
61–90 yr	
Male	13–40 units/L
Female	10–28 units/L
Greater than 90 yr	
Male	6–38 units/L
Female	5–24 units/L

Values may be slightly elevated in older adults due to the effects of medications and the presence of multiple chronic or acute diseases with or without muted symptoms.

DESCRIPTION: Alanine aminotransferase (ALT), formerly known as serum glutamic pyruvic transaminase (SGPT), is an enzyme produced by the liver. The highest concentration of ALT is found in liver cells; moderate amounts are found in kidney cells; and smaller amounts are found in heart, pancreas, spleen, skeletal muscle, and red blood cells. When liver damage occurs, serum levels of ALT rise to 50 times normal, making this a sensitive and useful test in evaluating liver injury.

INDICATIONS

• Compare serially with aspartate aminotransferase (AST) levels to track the course of liver disease
• Monitor liver damage resulting from hepatotoxic drugs
• Monitor response to treatment of liver disease, with tissue repair indicated by gradually declining levels

POTENTIAL DIAGNOSIS

Increased in
Related to release of ALT from damaged liver, kidney, heart, pancreas,
red blood cells, or skeletal muscle cells.
• Acute pancreatitis
• AIDS (related to hepatitis B co-infection)
• Biliary tract obstruction
• Burns (severe)
• Chronic alcohol abuse
• Cirrhosis
• Fatty liver
• Hepatic carcinoma
• Hepatitis
• Infectious mononucleosis
• Muscle injury from intramuscular injections, trauma, infection, and seizures (recent)
• Muscular dystrophy
• Myocardial infarction
• Myositis
• Pancreatitis
• Pre-eclampsia
• Shock (severe)

Decreased in
• Pyridoxal phosphate deficiency ***(related to a deficiency of pyridoxal phosphate that results in decreased production of ALT)***

CRITICAL FINDINGS: N/A

INTERFERING FACTORS
• Drugs that may increase ALT levels by causing cholestasis include

A

anabolic steroids, dapsone, estrogens, ethionamide, icterogenin, mepazine, methandriol, oral contraceptives, oxymetholone, propoxyphene, sulfonylureas, and zidovudine.

- Drugs that may increase ALT levels by causing hepatocellular damage include acetaminophen (toxic), acetylsalicylic acid, anticonvulsants, asparaginase, carbutamide, cephalosporins, chloramphenicol, clofibrate, cytarabine, danazol, dinitrophenol, enflurane, erythromycin, ethambutol, ethionamide, ethotoin, florantyrone, foscarnet, gentamicin, gold salts, halothane, ibufenac, indomethacin, interleukin-2, isoniazid, lincomycin, low-molecular-weight heparin, metahexamide, metaxalone, methoxsalen, methyldopa, methylthiouracil, naproxen, nitrofurans, oral contraceptives, probenecid, procainamide, and tetracyclines.
- Drugs that may decrease ALT levels include cyclosporine, interferons, metronidazole (affects enzymatic test methods), and ursodiol.

NURSING IMPLICATIONS AND PROCEDURE

PRETEST:

- Positively identify the patient using at least two unique identifiers before providing care, treatment, or services.
- *Patient Teaching:* Inform the patient this test can assist with evaluation of liver function and help identify disease.
- Obtain a history of the patient's complaints, including a list of known allergens, especially allergies or sensitivities to latex.
- Obtain a history of the patient's hepatobiliary system, symptoms, and results of previously performed laboratory tests and diagnostic and surgical procedures.

- Obtain a list of the patient's current medications including herbs, nutritional supplements, and nutraceuticals (see Appendix F).
- Review the procedure with the patient. Inform the patient that specimen collection takes approximately 5 to 10 min. Address concerns about pain and explain that there may be some discomfort during the venipuncture.
- *Sensitivity to social and cultural issues,* as well as concern for modesty, is important in providing psychological support before, during, and after the procedure.
- There are no food, fluid, or medication restrictions unless by medical direction.

INTRATEST:

- If the patient has a history of allergic reaction to latex, avoid the use of equipment containing latex.
- Instruct the patient to cooperate fully and to follow directions. Direct the patient to breathe normally and to avoid unnecessary movement.
- Observe standard precautions, and follow the general guidelines in Appendix A. Positively identify the patient, and label the appropriate specimen container with the corresponding patient demographics, initials of the person collecting the specimen, date, and time of collection. Perform a venipuncture.
- Remove the needle, and apply direct pressure with dry gauze to stop bleeding. Observe/assess venipuncture site for bleeding and hematoma formation and secure gauze with adhesive bandage.
- Promptly transport the specimen to the laboratory for processing and analysis.

POST-TEST:

- A report of the results will be made available to the requesting health-care provider (HCP), who will discuss the results with the patient.
- Instruct the patient to resume usual diet, fluids, medications, or activity, as directed by the HCP.

Nutritional Considerations: Increased ALT levels may be associated with liver disease. Dietary recommendations may be indicated and vary depending on the severity of the condition. A low-protein diet may be in order if the patient's liver has lost the ability to process the end products of protein metabolism. A diet of soft foods may be required if esophageal varices have developed. Ammonia levels may be used to determine whether protein should be added to or reduced from the diet. Patients should be encouraged to eat simple carbohydrates and emulsified fats (as in homogenized milk or eggs) rather than complex carbohydrates (e.g., starch, fiber, and glycogen [animal carbohydrates]) and complex fats, which require additional bile to emulsify them so that they can be used. The cirrhotic patient should be carefully observed for the development of ascites, in which case fluid and electrolyte balance requires strict attention.

Provide teaching and information regarding the clinical implications of the test results as appropriate. Educate the patient regarding access to counseling services. Provide contact information, if desired, for the Centers for Disease Control and Prevention (www.cdc.org/diseasesconditions).

Reinforce information given by the patient's HCP regarding further testing, treatment, or referral to another HCP. Answer any questions or address any concerns voiced by the patient or family.

Depending on the results of this procedure, additional testing may be performed to evaluate or monitor progression of the disease process and determine the need for a change in therapy. Evaluate test results in relation to the patient's symptoms and other tests performed.

RELATED MONOGRAPHS:

Related tests include acetaminophen, ammonia, AST, bilirubin, biopsy liver, cholangiography percutaneous transhepatic, electrolytes, GGT, hepatitis antigens and antibodies, LDH, liver and spleen scan, US abdomen, and US liver.

See the Hepatobiliary System table at the end of the book for related tests by body system.

Albumin and Albumin/Globulin Ratio

SYNONYM/ACRONYM: Alb, A/G ratio.

COMMON USE: To assess liver or kidney function and nutritional status.

SPECIMEN: Serum (1 mL) collected in a red- or tiger-top tube. Plasma (1 mL) collected in a green-top (heparin) tube is also acceptable.

NORMAL FINDINGS: (Method: Spectrophotometry) Normally the albumin/globulin (A/G) ratio is greater than 1.

A

Age	Conventional Units	SI Units (Conventional Units × 10)
Cord	2.8–4.3 g/dL	28–43 g/L
Newborn–7 d	2.6–3.6 g/dL	26–36 g/L
8–30 d	2.0–4.5 g/dL	20–45 g/L
1–3 mo	2.0–4.8 g/dL	20–48 g/L
4–6 mo	2.1–4.9 g/dL	21–49 g/L
7–12 mo	2.1–4.7 g/dL	21–47 g/L
1–3 yr	3.4–4.2 g/dL	34–42 g/L
4–6 yr	3.5–5.2 g/dL	35–52 g/L
7–19 yr	3.7–5.6 g/dL	37–56 g/L
20–40 yr	3.7–5.1 g/dL	37–51 g/L
41–60 yr	3.4–4.8 g/dL	34–48 g/L
61–90 yr	3.2–4.6 g/dL	32–46 g/L
Greater than 90 yr	2.9–4.5 g/dL	29–45 g/L

DESCRIPTION: Most of the body's total protein is a combination of albumin and globulins. Albumin, the protein present in the highest concentrations, is the main transport protein in the body. Albumin also significantly affects plasma oncotic pressure, which regulates the distribution of body fluid between blood vessels, tissues, and cells. Albumin is synthesized in the liver. Low levels of albumin may be the result of either inadequate intake, inadequate production, or excessive loss. Albumin levels are more useful as an indicator of chronic deficiency than of short-term deficiency.

Albumin levels are affected by posture. Results from specimens collected in an upright posture are higher than results from specimens collected in a supine position.

The albumin/globulin (A/G) ratio is useful in the evaluation of liver and kidney disease. The ratio is calculated using the following formula:

albumin/(total protein – albumin)

where globulin is the difference between the total protein value and the albumin value. For example, with a total protein of 7 g/dL and albumin of 4 g/dL, the A/G ratio is calculated as 4/(7 − 4) or 4/3 = 1.33. A reversal in the ratio, where globulin exceeds albumin (i.e., ratio less than 1.0), is clinically significant.

INDICATIONS
- Assess nutritional status of hospitalized patients, especially geriatric patients
- Evaluate chronic illness
- Evaluate liver disease

POTENTIAL DIAGNOSIS

Increased in
Any condition that results in a decrease of plasma water (e.g., dehydration); look for increase in hemoglobin and hematocrit. Decreases in the volume of intravascular liquid automatically result in concentration of the components present in the remaining liquid, as reflected by an elevated albumin level.
- Hyperinfusion of albumin

Decreased in
- *Insufficient intake:*
  Malabsorption *(related to lack of amino acids available for protein synthesis)*

A

Malnutrition *(related to insufficient dietary source of amino acids required for protein synthesis)*
* *Decreased synthesis by the liver:*
Acute and chronic liver disease (e.g., alcoholism, cirrhosis, hepatitis) *(evidenced by a decrease in normal liver function; the liver is the body's site of protein synthesis)*
Genetic analbuminemia *(related to genetic inability of liver to synthesize albumin)*
* *Inflammation and chronic diseases result in production of acute-phase reactant and other globulin proteins; the increase in globulins causes a corresponding decrease in albumin:*
Amyloidosis
Bacterial infections
Monoclonal gammopathies (e.g., multiple myeloma, Waldenström's macroglobulinemia)
Neoplasm
Parasitic infestations
Peptic ulcer
Prolonged immobilization
Rheumatic diseases
Severe skin disease
* *Increased loss over body surface:*
Burns *(evidenced by loss of interstitial fluid albumin)*
Enteropathies (e.g., gluten sensitivity, Crohn's disease, ulcerative colitis, Whipple's disease) *(evidenced by sensitivity to ingested substances or related to inadequate absorption from intestinal loss)*
Fistula (gastrointestinal or lymphatic) *(related to loss of sequestered albumin from general circulation)*
Hemorrhage *(related to fluid loss)*
Kidney disease *(related to loss from damaged renal tubules)*
Pre-eclampsia *(evidenced by excessive renal loss)*
Rapid hydration or overhydration *(evidenced by dilution effect)*
Repeated thoracentesis or paracentesis *(related to removal of albumin in accumulated third-space fluid)*

* *Increased catabolism:*
Cushing's disease *(related to excessive cortisol induced protein metabolism)*
Thyroid dysfunction *(related to overproduction of albumin binding thyroid hormones)*
* *Increased blood volume (hypervolemia):*
Congestive heart failure *(evidenced by dilution effect)*
Pre-eclampsia *(related to fluid retention)*
Pregnancy *(evidenced by increased circulatory volume from placenta and fetus)*

CRITICAL FINDINGS: N/A

INTERFERING FACTORS
* Drugs that may increase albumin levels include carbamazepine, furosemide, phenobarbital, and prednisolone.
* Drugs that may decrease albumin levels include acetaminophen (poisoning), amiodarone, asparaginase, dextran, estrogens, ibuprofen, interleukin-2, methotrexate, methyldopa, niacin, nitrofurantoin, oral contraceptives, phenytoin, prednisone, and valproic acid.
* Availability of administered drugs is affected by variations in albumin levels.

NURSING IMPLICATIONS AND PROCEDURE

PRETEST:
Positively identify the patient using at least two unique identifiers before providing care, treatment, or services.
Patient Teaching: Inform the patient this test can assist with evaluation of liver and kidney function, as well as chronic disease.
Obtain a history of the patient's complaints, including a list of known allergens, especially allergies or sensitivities to latex.

A

Obtain a history of the patient's gastrointestinal, genitourinary, and hepatobiliary systems; symptoms; and results of previously performed laboratory tests and diagnostic and surgical procedures.

Obtain a list of the patient's current medications including herbs, nutritional supplements, and nutraceuticals (see Appendix F).

Review the procedure with the patient. Inform the patient that specimen collection takes approximately 5 to 10 min. Address concerns about pain and explain that there may be some discomfort during the venipuncture.

Sensitivity to social and cultural issues, as well as concern for modesty, is important in providing psychological support before, during, and after the procedure.

There are no food, fluid, or medication restrictions unless by medical direction.

INTRATEST:

If the patient has a history of allergic reaction to latex, avoid the use of equipment containing latex.

Instruct the patient to cooperate fully and to follow directions. Direct the patient to breathe normally and to avoid unnecessary movement.

Observe standard precautions, and follow the general guidelines in Appendix A. Positively identify the patient, and label the appropriate specimen container with the corresponding patient demographics, initials of the person collecting the specimen, date, and time of collection. Perform a venipuncture.

Remove the needle and apply direct pressure with dry gauze to stop bleeding. Observe/assess venipuncture site for bleeding or hematoma formation and secure gauze with adhesive bandage.

Promptly transport the specimen to the laboratory for processing and analysis.

POST-TEST:

A report of the results will be made available to the requesting health-care provider (HCP), who will discuss the results with the patient.

Nutritional Considerations: Dietary recommendations may be indicated and will vary depending on the severity of the condition. Ammonia levels may be used to determine whether protein should be added to or reduced from the diet.

Reinforce information given by the patient's HCP regarding further testing, treatment, or referral to another HCP. Answer any questions or address any concerns voiced by the patient or family.

Depending on the results of this procedure, additional testing may be performed to evaluate or monitor progression of the disease process and determine the need for a change in therapy. Evaluate test results in relation to the patient's symptoms and other tests performed.

RELATED MONOGRAPHS:

Related tests include ALT, ALP, ammonia, anti–smooth muscle antibodies, AST, bilirubin, biopsy liver, CBC hematocrit, CBC hemoglobin, CT biliary tract and liver, GGT, hepatitis antibodies and antigens, KUB studies, laparoscopy abdominal, liver scan, MRI abdomen, osmolality, potassium, prealbumin, protein total and fractions, radiofrequency ablation liver, sodium, US abdomen, and US liver.

See the Gastrointestinal, Genitourinary, and Hepatobiliary systems tables at the end of the book for related tests by body system.

EDMUND CAMPION

A DEFINITIVE BIOGRAPHY